CAREERS IN
ANESTHESIOLOGY

Medical Doctor (MD)

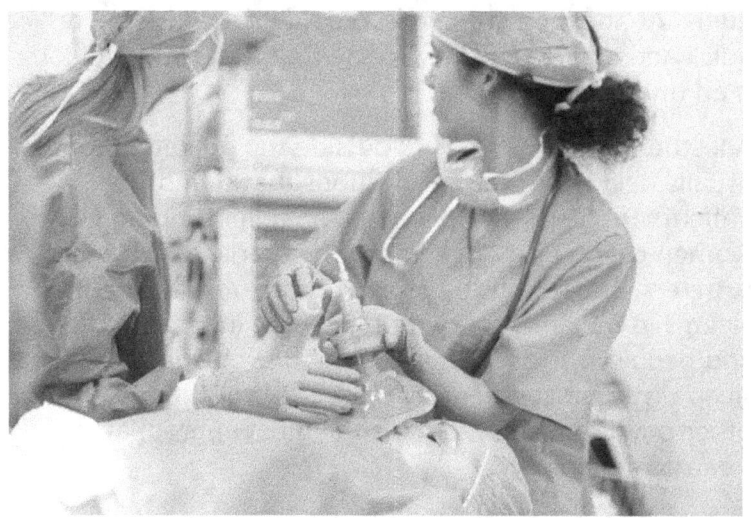

IN 1846, THE FIRST ANESTHETIC TO be successfully used for surgery was publicly demonstrated. Ether was immediately declared, "The greatest gift ever made to suffering humanity." Today's anesthetic drugs are different, but their importance has not lessened. It is the administration of safe and effective anesthesia that makes it possible for doctors to perform surgeries and other medical treatments that would otherwise kill their patients, or at least cause them great suffering.

Anesthesiologists are physicians who provide relief to patients in pain. In the operating room, they deliver anesthetic drugs, usually intravenously, that render people unconscious for the duration of the surgery. They may also deliver a sedative to keep the patient calm and relaxed. During the surgery, anesthesiologists work alongside surgeons, carefully monitoring a range of vital signs to make sure the patient is safe, comfortable, and pain-free. Sometimes it is necessary to adjust the amount of anesthetic, change the patient's position, or provide fluids. At any moment, a crisis could arise that requires quick action to save a life. To say that it is a stressful job is an understatement.

Anesthesiologists also work outside the operating room, usually delivering pain medications that do not put patients to sleep. They provide pain relief for pregnant women giving birth, patients with chronic pain, cancer sufferers, patients in the intensive care unit, accident victims in the emergency room, people in hospice care, and people who are suffering health problems due to sleep disturbances. In every case, they collaborate with other physicians to determine the most appropriate treatment plans.

Anesthesiology is a prestigious field that comes with a significant amount of responsibility. It also requires a great deal of education and expertise. It can take a minimum of 12 years of training to become a fully-fledged anesthesiologist! It starts with four years of undergraduate work followed by four years of medical school. Upon graduating from medical school, students will be an MD (Doctor of Medicine degree). Then comes the training in anesthesiology. That consists of a year in a general internship followed by three years of residency. After the residency is completed, they are eligible to sit for the national certification exams. However, many continue on to complete a year as a fellow, which provides for additional training in a specific field of anesthesiology, such as pediatrics, hospice and palliative medicine, obstetrics, cardiac care, critical care, or neuro-anesthesia. Certification is available in any of these sub-specialties.

In addition to an immense amount of medical knowledge, anesthesiologists must possess dexterity to insert IV lines and breathing tubes and use various specialized medical equipment. Other useful traits include empathy, strong communications skills, the ability to focus for extended periods, and being detail oriented.

Those who make it through the many years of training and preparation will find themselves in a particularly lucrative field of medicine. The median salary for anesthesiologists is well over $300,000 a year, which is even more than most surgeons make. Most are hired directly out of school because the demand for trained anesthesiologists is greater than the supply. Despite the obvious tangible rewards, most anesthesiologists (over 80 percent) report exceptional job satisfaction, but not because of the money or job security. They say they love their work because they spend their days making someone else's life better.

WHAT YOU CAN DO NOW

A RIGOROUS EDUCATION IS REQUIRED to become an anesthesiologist. High school students should prepare early and carefully to make sure all college entrance requirements are covered. At the very least that means four years each of math, English, and natural sciences. Biology is a must, along with chemistry and physics. Communications and a foreign language are important, too, since anesthesiologists talk to patients from all backgrounds. To prepare yourself for the rigors of the higher education ahead, develop good study habits and take challenging courses. AP (Advanced Placement) courses like chemistry, biology, and physics will look good to the college admissions office.

Learn as much as you can about this career to make sure it is the right choice for you. You can ask your guidance counselor to help set up a job shadow. You can also simply contact your local hospital and ask to talk to someone in anesthesiology. If you can talk to more than one, that is even better. Make the most of the opportunity to ask questions about their work, what to expect in school, and what they like and dislike about their work. Most of these professionals will be more than happy to show you around and share their experiences.

Get some first-hand experience in the healthcare field. It does not have to be directly related to anesthesiology to be of value. Ideally, you would find a part-time job in a hospital or dentist's office. If you cannot find a job, volunteer. Any position you can get will help you determine if healthcare is your calling. Plus, it will look good on your college entrance application.

HISTORY OF THE CAREER

OF ALL THE ACHIEVEMENTS IN MEDICINE throughout history, none is more important than the introduction of anesthetics. When the first anesthetic for use in surgery was successfully tested in the late 19th century, it was proclaimed the greatest gift ever made to suffering humanity. Until then, there had been many efforts to relieve pain throughout the ages. Some of the earliest involved crude and brutal attempts to induce unconsciousness by hitting the patient's head or by squeezing the carotid arteries in the neck. Unconsciousness was achieved in the Middle Ages with elaborate concoctions of alcohol and plant extracts like mandrake root. Another potion known as dwale was considered an advance, with its mixture of opium, hemlock, bile, bryony, and lettuce. It was used until the 16th century. Opium was eventually segregated and widely used, and the first intravenous injection of opium was made in the 1660s.

During the late 18th and early 19th centuries, much more research and experimentation were done with various gases and their effect on the heart and lungs. In 1799, nitrous oxide was the first of these gases to be employed for pain relief. Fifty years later, it was used during the extraction of teeth for the first time.

In 1825, English physician and promoter of anesthesia, Henry Hill Hickman, wrote about his experiments with carbon dioxide. He used the gas to induce "suspended animation" (loss of consciousness) in small animals and performed surgery on them. He reported in a treatise to the Royal Society that the animals seemed to feel no pain. This might have been an exciting breakthrough, but his findings were ignored and no drug was used for general anesthesia in humans until 20 years later. That drug was ether.

The first public demonstration of ether anesthesia for surgery was performed by dentist, Dr. William Morton, in Boston on October 16, 1846. This date is considered a major turning point and the beginning of the modern anesthetic era. Dr. Morton, along with renowned surgeon, John Warren, made history by proving that when ether is inhaled in the proper dose, it provided a safe and effective anesthesia. Recognizing the importance of the event, Massachusetts General Hospital named its operating room the Ether Dome, and it is preserved intact to this day. The news that the pain of surgery had been eliminated spread like wildfire around the world, and Dr. Morton was credited with being the founder of modern anesthesia. A few weeks after the famous demonstration, Oliver Wendell Holmes popularized the word "anesthesia" and introduced related terms like "anesthetic state" and "anesthetic agent."

Other forms of anesthesia were soon introduced. There were general forms like chloroform and the regional type like nerve blocks produced with cocaine. Various delivery methods were introduced, such as spinal cord injections and epidurals. Safety issues were noted when the first anesthetic death occurred in 1848 from the use of chloroform. In London, the famous Dr. John Snow led the way in analyzing complications after anesthesia and reviewing procedures.

By the late 1930s, general anesthesia became more pleasant for patients with the introduction of gases that allowed for a lighter depth of general anesthesia. The harsh and riskier agents like ether and chloroform eventually disappeared from operating rooms.

The Profession Emerges

Anesthesiology began as a trade rather than a true profession. It lacked important elements of professionalism, such as standards of care, innovations in clinical science, rigorous educational programs, and professional organizations to support research and distribute information. For a time, it was nurses, rather than doctors, who administered anesthetics. It was not until the turn of the 20th century that doctors accepted this responsibility, and physician anesthetists gradually gained recognition. Starting in the very early 1900s, accomplished doctors became professors of anesthesia in medical schools and chiefs of anesthesia in hospitals. Still, professionalism was elusive.

In 1927, the University of Wisconsin tasked anesthesiologist Ralph Milton Waters with creating a separate department for anesthesiology. Professor Waters, who had contributed several significant inventions to the anesthetic field, considered the condition of the profession primitive. At the time, there were no professional societies and very few journals on the subject. He determined that in order for anesthesiology to become a true and respected profession, there needed to be high-level training programs, organizations to establish and oversee standards of education and practice, and support for research programs. He established a rigorous three-year residency program in Madison that produced numerous anesthesia department heads.

Waters's vision of bringing professionalism into the practice of anesthesia became a reality. Professional societies were formed, bringing best practices to the field. The accreditation process was initiated. Formal training programs were based on widely accepted standards, and academic departments devoted to anesthesia multiplied.

The Modern Era of Anesthesia

The second wave of rapid advances in anesthesia began in the 1960s. New drugs and equipment were developed. Drugs like sodium thiopental (pentothal) and propofol provided substantially shorter recovery time. Delivery systems and monitoring techniques were refined and safety came into sharp focus. Anesthesia led the way for the routine study and analysis of close calls, known as "critical incidents." It became possible to perform surgery on more complex procedures that might have been impossible before.

As we entered the information age at the end of the 20th century, anesthesiologists could receive relevant information from around the world faster and more efficiently. They learned of major advances that could improve their techniques and results, from microelectronics to tailoring anesthesia to each individual patient.

Today, advances in medicine like genetics and nano-technology, that could not have been dreamed of only a few decades ago, are being quickly integrated into the mainstream. Such rapid evolution portends an excellent future for anesthesia as well. Leaders in the field predict further improvements in monitors, protocols, education, and the analysis of Big Data that will make anesthesia safer than ever. While there will always be extremely difficult and challenging clinical situations, as well as human error, safety statistics show that anesthesia mortality and morbidity are rare and are becoming rarer. Anesthesia makes all surgical treatments and cures possible. That is the one fact that will not change.

WHERE YOU WILL WORK

THERE ARE CURRENTLY 45,000 ANESTHESIOLOGY JOBS in the US. They are located in a variety of settings. The most common are hospitals and outpatient surgical centers, but anesthesiologists also work in private physician offices, medical clinics, and military medical centers. Academic and medical institutions also need anesthesiologists to teach the necessary skills to students.

Some anesthesiologists operate private practices, usually within a group practice, although that is less common in this field than in most other physician specializations. Most anesthesiologists prefer to work in the hospital environment because it offers variety. The areas where anesthesiology is practiced has expanded dramatically in recent years. The operating room is still the most common place for anesthesiologists to work, but hospitals also need their expertise for invasive radiology, gastrointestinal endoscopy, electrophysiology, and other modern procedures.

The skills used in anesthesiology are basically the same in any job, but there are some subtle differences depending on where an anesthesiologist chooses to work. For example, one might have developed a delicate approach to anesthesiology that would be very welcome in healthcare clinics that mostly serve the elderly.

Due to the high demand for anesthesiologists, there are many new opportunities to travel as locum tenens practitioners. Locum tenens are temporary positions that may last a few weeks to several months. The jobs are located in all parts of the country, which gives adventurous anesthesiologists the chance to experience different locations and work in some of the best medical facilities.

Wherever anesthesiologists are located, they work in sterile, well-lit environments equipped with the latest devices and technology. Many anesthesiologists work long hours. This is especially true for those who work in hospitals where shifts are usually 12 hours long followed by 24 hours on call. However, anesthesiologists are rarely called when on call. More often than not, being on call means being at home. Although the hospital schedule still exists, there is a trend toward more normal eight-hour shifts. That is because more hospitals and other medical facilities are being taken over by corporations that prefer all their corporate employees to be scheduled the same way.

THE WORK YOU WILL DO

AN ANESTHESIOLOGIST IS A MEDICAL DOCTOR who specializes in administering medications or other medical methods to control pain. This typically means keeping a patient comfortable, safe and pain free during surgery. It is a key role in the operating room. Without properly delivered anesthesia, surgeons and other physicians would not be able to perform surgery or other invasive procedures on patients. Anesthesiologists work side-by-side with surgeons, making sure patients are stable and feel no pain throughout the procedure. They are responsible for maintaining the patient's critical life functions, which sometimes means making quick decisions on limited information.

For most surgeries, patients need to be placed in the controlled state of unconsciousness. It is what most people describe as being put to sleep, going under, or being knocked out. It is what anesthesiologists refer to as general anesthesia, which is similar to a powerful (but temporary) drug-induced coma. It is not the administration of a single drug, but rather a combination of carefully selected intravenous drugs and inhaled gasses. When a patient is having surgery on the head, chest, or abdomen, anesthesiologists also have to support a patient's breathing with a breathing tube.

General anesthesia is not always necessary. Anesthesiologists also utilize regional anesthetics, where only a part of the body is made numb. They may also administer sedation intravenously to relieve pain or anxiety and keep a patient calm. Regional anesthesia is usually administered differently than general anesthesia. Instead of delivering medications intravenously, anesthesiologists inject them near a knot of nerves to prevent pain signals from traveling to the brain. In effect, it numbs the nearby part of the body – or so the mind would believe. This is done while patients are awake, though they may be drowsy or even fall asleep after being sedated.

Operating Room Procedure

While it may appear that an anesthesiologist's job is only about rendering people unconscious for surgery, they are in fact responsible for much more than that. Every surgery begins with meeting the patient to conduct preoperative assessments. At this time, the anesthesiologist will take a thorough patient history and carefully review existing records with the patient, as well as assess the patient's current state of overall health. The doctor asks specific questions about any previous experiences with anesthesia and looks for any indication of allergic or other adverse reactions. The purpose of this evaluation process is to make sure that the patient is suitably prepared and medically fit to endure the planned surgery and the necessary anesthetic. Based on the information gathered, the anesthesiologist will develop the safest anesthesia plan, using the most appropriate medications for that individual patient.

Before surgery begins, the anesthesiology care team prepares the medications, delivery systems, and monitoring equipment. From the moment the patient enters the operating room, the anesthesiologist is alongside the patient, talking to the patient reassuringly and making sure they are comfortable and safe. Sedation is administered first to ensure that the patient is fully relaxed. Then just before surgery, the anesthetic is delivered, using local, intravenous, spinal, or caudal methods.

Throughout the surgery, anesthesiologists will closely monitor the patient's vital signs and critical life functions. They continually watch the patient's blood pressure inside the lung vessels, heart rhythm, temperature, level of consciousness, and amount of oxygen in the blood. For a general anesthetic, the anesthesiologist will monitor each breath by measuring the volume of breath exhaled and the amount of carbon dioxide in each breath. All the while, the anesthesiologist remains sharply focused and ready to counteract any adverse reactions or complications from the anesthesia or the surgery itself.

There are many details to attend to. For example, keeping patients warm in the cold operating room, providing the fluids their bodies need, padding their arms and legs and other pressure points, and adjusting their position as necessary. These are all important for the well-being and safety of the patient. Even something as simple as the position of the legs is important. Crossed legs during surgery can potentially cause nerve damage.

The anesthesiologist's job does not end when surgery is completed. The responsibility of maintaining a patient's health and safety continues until they wake up and recover from the effects of anesthetic medications.

Outside the Operating Room

The anesthesiologist's role extends beyond the operating room. They may be needed to control severe pain after a surgical procedure. They may be responsible for managing chronic pain, or the pain associated with cancer. They may work in emergency rooms, providing immediate pain relief or sedation as needed. They may also administer pain medications during blood transfusion therapies, respiratory therapy, and cardiac or respiratory resuscitation. Patients experience pain for many reasons, including burns, diabetes, herpes, migraines, or severe injuries from car accidents or other accidents. They may have pain in any area of their body. It requires the expertise of an anesthesiologist to correctly determine the safest, most effective method for controlling the pain over a period of hours, days, weeks, or even months.

Some anesthesiologists rarely, if ever, step foot inside an operating room. Instead, they choose to specialize in other areas of pain management, such as pediatrics, oncology, or chronic pain management. They may become board certified in one of a number of sub-specialties, including critical care medicine, hospice and palliative medicine, pain medicine for outpatient chronic or cancer pain, pediatric medicine, and sleep medicine. Critical care specialists are based in the intensive care unit (ICU) of a hospital. Specialists in hospice and palliative medicine work to prevent and relieve the suffering of patients with life-limiting illnesses. Pain medicine anesthesiologists work with outpatient chronic or cancer pain. Pediatric specialists work exclusively with neonates, infants, children, and adolescents undergoing painful surgical, diagnostic, or therapeutic procedures. Sleep specialists are skilled in the diagnosis and management of clinical conditions that occur during sleep. One of the most common types of specialization is obstetrics. Obstetrical anesthesiologists help manage pain during childbirth.

The Anesthesia Care Team

Like most types of healthcare, anesthesia requires teamwork. The anesthesiologist is the director of the anesthesia care team, which may include two non-physician professionals: an anesthesiology assistant and a nurse anesthetist.

An anesthesiologist assistant (AA) is a highly skilled and certified health professional who has completed an accredited four-year degree that satisfies pre-med requirements. Their job is to act as an extension of the anesthesiologist, performing important tasks that allow the anesthesiologist to focus on administering medications and maintaining life support to surgical patients. Typical tasks may include taking health histories, performing physical exams, taking blood, pre-testing and calibrating anesthesia delivery systems and monitors, ensuring continuity of care through the postoperative recovery period, performing administrative duties, and assisting with life support as required. They are also able to help with preparatory procedures like pulmonary artery catheterization or echocardiography. AAs are only allowed to practice within the field of anesthesia, under the direct supervision of an anesthesiologist.

A Certified Registered Nurse Anesthetist (CRNA) is a registered nurse who has earned a master's degree, plus completed two to three years of additional training in the field of patient assessment, pain control, and patient recovery services. Although they are not physicians, their training is similar to that of anesthesiologists. They are often supervised by an anesthesiologist, but they also work under the supervision of other types of doctors. Unlike AAs, they are relatively independent, and may administer anesthesia during surgical, therapeutic, diagnostic, and obstetric procedures. In fact, CRNAs administer about over 40 million anesthetics each year in the US. In addition to administering anesthetics, they perform nerve blocks, monitor vital signs during medical procedures, and provide pre-op and post-op care.

CRNAs usually work in hospital operating rooms, emergency rooms, intensive care units, cardiac care units, outpatient surgical clinics, military medical facilities, and mobile surgery centers. They may also work in the offices of dentists, ophthalmologists, plastic surgeons, podiatrists, and chronic pain management specialists.

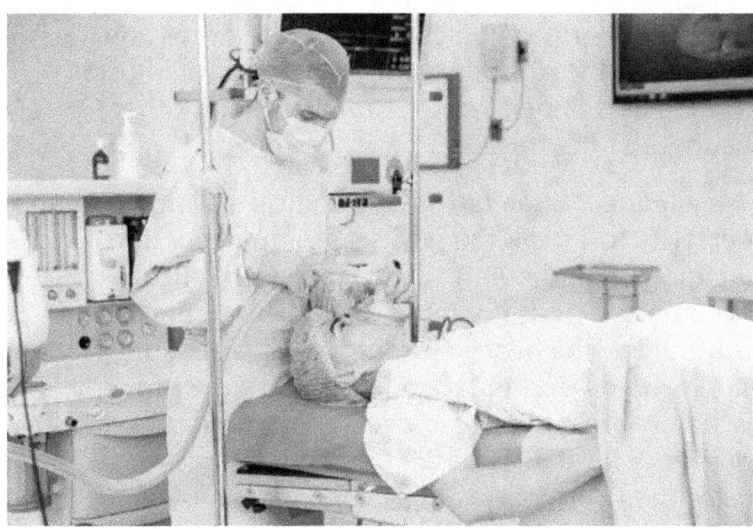

STORIES OF THESE DOCTORS AT WORK

I Specialize in Critical Care

"I provide anesthesia for patients who undergo surgery and other invasive procedures, often under emergency conditions. It is very intellectually challenging work. I have to be ready to recognize heart or lung problems that may complicate the patient's surgery, and judge which medications are appropriate. All anesthesiologists are trained to understand the complex pharmacologic effects of the drugs and determine the right dose, how to program infusion devices and understand the monitors and other gadgets of the trade.

Knowledge is vital, but so is technical skill and manual dexterity to use all the devices, pumps, monitors, and imaging equipment. It takes years of practice to become skilled at finding veins that sometimes lead centrally to the heart in order to deliver the medication safely. If you don't place a breathing tube properly, an ischemic brain injury can occur within minutes. If the dose of a local anesthetic for an epidural isn't calculated correctly, cardiac collapse can happen within seconds. If the anesthesiologist loses focus during an aortic aneurysm case, a patient can bleed out in the time it takes to cross an operating room floor.

Anesthesiologists are sometimes compared to pilots. No one applauds when the plane lands safely, and likewise, everyone expects a perfect, uncomplicated anesthetic experience every time. What people don't see when an anesthesiologist is sitting calmly and quietly at the head of the operating table is the intense concentration on a myriad of details that could mean the difference between life and death. It is intense work and to say it is stressful would be an understatement. It is the kind of work where if you are having a bad day, you still have to perform at your best. Some people thrive under that kind of pressure. Those who don't should probably choose a different field of medicine."

I Focus on High-Risk Inpatient Cases

"I enjoy the challenges of complex cases, like high-risk obstetrics, level I trauma (the most serious), or thoracic surgery where I've only got one lung to ventilate. As long as I have my resuscitation drugs, monitors, blood products, bronchoscopes, and other tools, I am perfectly happy to take on the sickest patient in the hospital.

It takes a certain type of person to enjoy this kind of work. You have to be able to handle routine and predictable tasks without losing focus, while at the same time be ready to jump into action when crises arise. There is no time to deliberate at length before taking action. On the other hand, there is immediate gratification. When I deliver medication through the patient's IV, I know immediately if it worked like I planned. I don't have to wait until the next office visit to see the results.

You also have to be okay with not knowing what time you will be going home. It is sometimes impossible to predict how long a surgery will take. High level trauma facilities like mine require anesthesiologists in house 24/7, with 12 hour shifts and several overnights each month.

The good news is there are options for those who really want to go into anesthesiology, but don't really like being based in the operating room, or even in a hospital. I suggest looking at all the possibilities, and choosing clinical rotations in medical school in as many specialty areas as you can. Don't try to pick your specialization too soon. You won't really know what field is right for you until you make your way through those rotations."

I Work in Orthopedics

"When I was in medical school, I wasn't sure what field I would go into. My strong interest in sports had me leaning toward sports medicine. With that in mind, I shadowed an orthopedist at an outpatient orthopedic clinic. Part of that experience allowed me to spend a day in the operating room watching knee arthroscopies. I was fascinated with the technical aspects of the procedure and loved the orderliness of the OR. There was a rhythm to it with cases being scheduled, patients anesthetized, procedures completed, and patients discharged. That was when I realized that chronic care would test my patience. In a clinic situation, I would see a patient, write a prescription, and the patient would leave. Until the patient returned weeks later, I wouldn't know if the prescription was actually filled, if there were undesirable side effects, or if the treatment was working at all. I prefer knowing the outcome of my medical care as soon as I deliver it.

As it happened, I wasn't able to talk to the orthopedic

surgeon that day. Rather, I ended up standing next to the anesthesiologist who talked to me about his career choice between patients. He explained some of the things he was doing and I became intrigued with how the pharmacology controlled the physiology of the body. He also impressed upon me the need for empathy. Every surgical patient is in a battle with an illness or disease. Even though anesthesiologists only see the patient for a few minutes before surgery, they can have a profound impact on the outcome. Many medical students are attracted to anesthesiology for the money and job security, but unless you truly want to help the people in your care, you won't be happy in this field. Today, in those few minutes before my patient is wheeled into the OR, I try to reassure them at what may be the scariest moment of their lives."

PERSONAL QUALIFICATIONS

ANESTHESIOLOGISTS PLAY A VITAL ROLE in the operating room, one that is equal to the surgeon. Getting to this prestigious position takes many years of hard work and training. Years of memorizing facts about physiology, pharmacology, and disease are a good start, but it requires more than medical knowledge to thrive. Besides being extremely smart people, anesthesiologists share several personal characteristics that help them achieve successful surgeries and recoveries. The first is a strong desire to help people. Like every other physician, anesthesiologists must care about each individual patient. That empathy must start with the first contact before surgery and continue on throughout surgery and into the recovery room.

Because anesthesiologists have little time to interact with patients, especially in emergency situations, they need superior communication and interpersonal skills. They typically have less than 10 minutes to establish rapport, conduct an examination, obtain consent, and gain trust. This is not an easy feat when patients are naturally anxious about having surgery. In addition to managing their medical needs, you have to address their emotional needs. This can be accomplished with a calm, reassuring voice that explains in clear terms what to expect.

Anesthesiologists do not work alone. Collaboration with other medical personnel is essential. During surgery, you have to work effectively with all types of surgeons regardless of their personalities, which are often seen as egotistical or brusque. Outside the operating room, anesthesiologists may find themselves in the delivery room, intensive care unit, or emergency room. They must work well together with teams of nurses, medical techs, internists, obstetricians, family practitioners, and respiratory therapists to provide pain management for all types of chronic and acute pain.

Physical stamina and a tolerance for fatigue are necessary. Scheduled surgeries often start at 7:30am and the anesthesiologist has to start before that time to meet with the patient, get them to the operating room, and render them unconscious. Surgeries can continue throughout the day and emergency surgeries can occur at any time of the day or night. The anesthesiologist must remain focused and attentive at all times.

Manual dexterity is also needed. It takes a steady hand and an agile touch to insert a spinal catheter or breathing tube, inject a nerve block near peripheral nerves, or administer an epidural. It is not uncommon for aspiring anesthesiologists to drop out of the specialty because they are unable to consistently conduct these procedures with ease.

An anesthesiologist's job is one of the most stressful of all medical specialties. Imagine your patient, helpless and unconscious on the operating table. Suddenly their heart rate drops dangerously low, their blood pressures spikes, they hemorrhage from an artery, or they cannot breathe. These moments can and do happen. In these life-threatening events, it is imperative that the anesthesiologist remain calm and decisive. Successful anesthesiologists rely on their training and clinical judgment to make the correct diagnostic and therapeutic moves swiftly while under intense pressure.

ATTRACTIVE FEATURES

ANESTHESIOLOGISTS MAKE A LIVING putting people to sleep, but this specialty is anything but dull. Anesthesiologists describe it as the most interesting job in the world, with more perks than other doctors receive. It is fast-paced and intellectually challenging, yet accommodating to family life. The high-pressure workdays are offset by plentiful personal time. In their work environment, the operating room, they play a pivotal role that is vital to successful outcomes. The allure of this career may be high pay, but there are multiple reasons anesthesiologists are happy with their choice.

It is no secret that anesthesiologists enjoy excellent pay. It has been ranked the #1 best paying job in America by US News & World Report. It pays more than other medical specialties, sometimes even topping a surgeon's pay. One medical professional association's survey found that the median annual income (salary plus bonus) for anesthesiologists was over $440,000, versus $407,000 for surgeons. That explains why there is so much competition for spots in anesthesiology residency programs.

It takes a long time to become an anesthesiologist, but once you have paid your dues you can count on finding a good job. The job growth has been exceptionally strong for many years, and there is no sign of decline in the foreseeable future. Due to the high demand for anesthesiologists, job security is outstanding. It is unusual for a career to last a lifetime these days, but it is common for anesthesiologists to practice well into their 70s. Occasionally anesthesiologists experience career burnout, but it has been less frequent than in other high-stress medical specialties like surgery and emergency medicine.

Anesthesiologists enjoy more flexibility than most other medical professionals. They have many practice options without having to maintain their own office. They can join the staff of a hospital or other medical center, practice at an outpatient surgery center, with a group administering office-based anesthesia, or practice pain management in an office setting. Even in the most common setting, the hospital, there are choices. For example, they can work exclusively in the operating room, run intensive care units, or be an on-call locum tenens.

Most anesthesiologists work full time, but there is some flexibility. Outside the hospital environment, it is possible to control your schedule, making it shorter and more consistent. Because the skills and procedures are almost the same in every practice environment, it is easy to have someone cover for you if you need time off without disrupting the surgical schedule. Even in the hospital environment, where attending anesthesiologists often work long 12-hour shifts, there are plenty of paid days (PTO) and vacation time to create a balanced lifestyle.

Immediate gratification is not part of the typical doctor's experience. Controlling the body's functions is a quick process that are accomplished in a matter of hours or even just minutes. The procedure may be brief, but it can also be intense. Controlling a patient's breathing, circulation, and airway and watching the changes in real time are exciting for those who are well prepared. It appeals to those who are results driven and like to see the outcome of their work without waiting. That is the essence of acute care. Most anesthesiologists would be bored with chronic care, where treatment with each patient can go on for days, weeks, months, or even years. Doctors who choose acute care thrive on the fast pace and knowing that thrilling things may happen at any moment.

UNATTRACTIVE ASPECTS

DESPITE THE MANY BENEFITS THAT COME with being an anesthesiologist, there are challenges that should be considered. The first hurdle is to get through 10 years of schooling. The requirements to enter the profession are strict and the field is extremely popular. Even assuming the student has an aptitude for medicine and is an excellent student, there is tough competition for residency positions.

Anesthesiology is one of the most stressful jobs in medicine. It is fast-paced, yet the anesthesiologist must be laser-focused on every detail. When a patient is on the operating table, a life is literally in the hands of the anesthesiologist and the surgeon. Failing to pay attention even for a second, can have disastrous results. For example, if the anesthesiologist forgets to insert a breathing tube, brain death could occur in minutes. Or if a patient has an allergic reaction to the anesthetic agent, the heart can stop. The anesthesiologist must be well-prepared and alert, ready to jump into action and save a life.

Workloads can be heavy. Anesthesiologists are needed at all hours in hospitals and emergency care facilities. Some surgeries take longer than anticipated, forcing the workday to extend into overtime.

While it is good that anesthesiologists are in demand, the downside is packed schedules that start before most of us have enjoyed our first cup of coffee. If everything goes smoothly, they may be home in time for dinner, but an emergency surgery or an add-on patient can mean working around the clock.

Anesthesiologists are exposed to numerous bacteria, viruses, and other pathogens. There are risks for both airborne and bloodborne infections that may be contracted while securing intravenous lines, through needle sticks during suturing of central venous catheters, or other points of exposure to the patient's body fluids. Anesthesiologists are trained to avoid these hazards through strict safety procedures.

Radiation is a potential hazard to anesthesiologists. The anesthesiologist is exposed to radiation much more often than other medical professionals during certain procedures. The use of C-arm (mobile imaging) is on the rise, exposing anesthesiologists to radiation beyond the recommended dose limit. The cumulative effects of radiation can affect the entire body or cause localized damage to a certain area of the body such as cataracts in the eyes. Following safety procedures to the letter can reduce the risk significantly.

EDUCATION AND TRAINING

BECOMING AN ANESTHESIOLOGIST IS NOT EASY. It takes at least 12 years to complete the education and training required to become fully qualified to practice in this medical specialty. It starts with four years of undergraduate studies, followed by four years of medical school, a one-year internship (sometimes called a transitional or preliminary year), and three years of residency specializing in anesthesiology.

Although not required, most anesthesiology residents continue their training for an additional year in a fellowship program that will prepare them for a subspecialty, such as pain management, cardiac anesthesiology, pediatric anesthesiology, neuro-anesthesiology, obstetric anesthesiology or critical care medicine. Along the way, there are admissions tests and competency exams at every stage.

The first step is to earn a bachelor's degree. Students can major in any field, but it is vital that they build a strong foundation in biology, chemistry, and physics. An emphasis should also be placed on mathematics and English. The best way to ensure that you are prepared is to enroll in a pre-med bachelor's degree program. Not all schools offer this and it is possible to put together your own version with the help of a guidance counselor.

Medical School

Medical school is hard work – hard to get in and hard to stay in. Only students with exceptional academic records can expect to be admitted. The American Medical Association (AMA) reports that successful applicants typically have a college GPA of 3.5-4.0, but admission is not based on grades alone. Students must have demonstrated their sincere dedication to a future in medicine through clinical or healthcare experience. That typically consists of volunteer work in a clinic or hospital. A bonus benefit to these experiences is the opportunity to gather letters of recommendation from doctors and other healthcare professionals.

The final requirement to get into medical school is a passing score on the Medical College Admission Test (MCAT). There are three parts to the MCAT: biological sciences, verbal reasoning, and physical sciences. Multiple choice questions will cover subjects like physics, biology, and organic and general chemistry, and critical thinking. Unlike admissions tests in other fields, the essay requirement has been dropped. Students can prepare for the MCAT through the Association of American Medical Colleges (AAMC). The organization offers content outlines for each part, an official guide, and practice tests. There is a charge for these resources, but most students consider it well worth the investment.

The first year of medical school consists of courses in the basic sciences. The second year focuses on organ systems. Clinical training starts In the third year. Students move through a series of clinical rotations where they learn to diagnose and treat a variety of patients. In the fourth year, they are able to choose their rotations based on their own interests. There are usually four-week rotations to fulfill training requirements. During this time, students preparing for a residency in anesthesia have the opportunity to work alongside anesthesiologists who can further educate them in patient care and techniques.

Aspiring anesthesiologists should be continually preparing for the United States Medical Licensing Examination (USMLE) while in medical school. All doctors must pass this exam to become licensed to practice medicine in the US. There are three steps to the USMLE. The first two can be taken during medical school or after graduation. The third cannot be taken until after receiving an MD degree.

Residency

Upon graduating medical school, students earn an MD degree. Now they are eligible to participate in a residency program. The first year involves completing various hospital rotations. Anesthesiology residents can spend the following three years in clinical anesthesia (CA) training. CA training starts out with basic instruction on the fundamental principles of anesthesia. This is followed by rotations related to anesthesia subspecialties, including cardiac anesthesia, pediatric anesthesia, and regional anesthesia. For the last two years of CA training, residents can choose between advanced clinical training or clinical research.

State Licensing

Like all physicians, anesthesiologists must apply for licensing through the medical board in the state where they plan to practice. In addition to holding a medical degree and completing residency training, they must pass practical and written exams. At this stage, they must also pass the third and final step of the USMLE for national medical licensing.

Board Certification

Although board certification is not a requirement, most employers expect anesthesiologists to be board certified. It demonstrates advanced skill and knowledge and using the title of Board Certified Anesthesiologist can help with opening the door to more opportunities or put the doctor in a good position to negotiate for a higher salary. Most choose to receive their certification through the American Board of Anesthesiology (ABA). The American Board of Physician Specialties (ABPS) also offers a similar process. In addition to the basic certification, the ABA offers certification options in subspecialties that include critical care medicine, pain medicine, hospice and palliative medicine, sleep medicine, and pediatric anesthesiology.

EARNINGS

ADMINISTERING ANESTHESIA IS A HIGHLY responsible job that requires a decade of professional training. As a result, anesthesiologists are paid well, typically more than $300,000 a year. Note that salaries for anesthesiologists, unlike most occupations, have risen substantially in recent years. Salaries have increased 20 percent on average. With the current heavy demand for these professionals, it is expected that salaries will continue to rise.

The median annual salary is $375,000, with a range between $350,000 and $425,000. Since this is a median, half of anesthesiologists earn even more. The American Medical Group Association, a reliable source of physicians' salaries, reports the median income for anesthesiologists at $440,000. Why the difference? It is because the Association's survey includes total compensation, including bonuses. Bonuses are common in this field and can add as much as $75,000 on top of the base salary.

Compared to other medical specialties, anesthesiologists are the clear winners in high earnings. Surgeons are in second place with a median annual compensation of $400,000 and pediatrics looks meager by comparison at only $228,000.

Although all anesthesiologists do well, earnings will vary by geographic location, number of years in practice, type of employment, and professional reputation. In general, however, more money is earned by those who are somewhat independent. For example, as a salaried employee, an anesthesiologist would earn an average of $350,000 a year. With the same level of experience and skills, that same anesthesiologist who is a partner in private practice can expect an average income of $400,000.

Anesthesiologists working through locum tenens agencies do even better, with a nationwide average annual salary of $440,000. That works out to more than $36,500 per month, which is especially good considering these professionals can pick and choose when and where they work and rarely put in the total hours that salaried employees do. Their compensation is bolstered by bonuses, travel expenses, and housing subsidies.

OPPORTUNITIES

THERE ARE CURRENTLY 45,000 ANESTHESIOLOGY JOBS in the US. The number of jobs is expected to grow by almost 20 percent over the coming decade, which amounts to another 5,900 new jobs opening up in the near future. This is a faster rate of job growth than for most other healthcare occupations.

One of the driving forces behind the increased demand for anesthesiologists is the aging population, which is continuing to grow as most baby boomers are past retirement age. As people get older, the likelihood of necessary surgeries and chronic illnesses rises. There is also a need for pain relief during the more challenging diagnostic tests and therapies. Anesthesiologists are often called upon to help make patients in hospice as comfortable as possible.

The high demand for skilled anesthesiologists has resulted in an unemployment rate of less than one percent. An increasing number of medical students are attracted to the specialty for a variety of reasons – high pay, lighter patient load, prestige, and intriguing technology, to name a few. Additional anesthesiology residents would seem to solve the problem of supply versus demand. However, residency programs in anesthesiology are extremely competitive and many aspiring anesthesiologists are turned away and end up pursuing other areas of specialized practice.

Those who are smart enough and can handle the extremely hard work to make it through training, will find that many opportunities exist for anesthesiologists of all skill levels. Most are placed in their first jobs immediately after graduating. The prospects are especially good for those who are willing to work in rural or low-income areas that have difficulty attracting medical personnel. Newly licensed anesthesiologists have options – they can choose where they want to work and what type of environment they would prefer.

The scope of the profession has expanded greatly over the past 10 years. The majority of these doctors still work in hospital operating rooms, but their expertise is now needed in other places. For example, anesthesiology is a necessary procedure in gastrointestinal endoscopy, electrophysiology, and invasive radiology. Some anesthesiologists work in intensive care units where they help stabilize critically ill or injured patients. Others work in oncology departments to help manage the pain of cancer patients or work with hematologists during blood transfusion therapies. Wherever an anesthesiologist wants to work, the doctor needs to build a reputation for working well within a team. That reputation alone can open many more doors.

There is particularly heavy demand for anesthesiologists in locum placements agencies. These agencies place anesthesiologists in temporary assignments, usually outside their home town. This is an especially good option for those who are undecided about where and how they want to work. Most of these traveling professionals are covering for staff anesthesiologists who are on vacation, maternity leave, sick leave, or hiatus. Many assignments are with the country's best medical facilities. The skills in this field are virtually the same for any position, making any situation easy to step into and less intimidating than many other types of temp jobs. One of the benefits of this is the opportunity to gain experience and quickly build a good reputation for being a valued team player.

GETTING STARTED

YOU SHOULD LAY THE GROUNDWORK for your first job search during your residency. Your first stop will be the school's career center. New job listings will be posted as they come up and there will be notices of recruiters scheduled to visit. There are other valuable services, too. For example, creating a strong résumé and cover letter may not be your forte. At the career center, you can get help writing a résumé that will stand out to potential employers and also practice your interviewing techniques.

Make a daily habit of searching the internet for jobs. It is by far the fastest and most practical resource available for anesthesiologists. You can go to the general job sites like Indeed and Glassdoor that make it easy to look for jobs that meet your criteria for location, salary, and experience level. There are also several job sites devoted entirely to helping anesthesiologists find jobs. For example, GasWork.com allows you to browse postings from healthcare centers across the country and you can easily submit your cover letter and résumé through the site. It is so quick and easy, you can apply for multiple jobs the same day.

There are employment agencies that specialize in healthcare jobs, both online and off. Some only handle full-time permanent positions, usually within their local area. Others handle locum tenens situations, which means temporarily taking the place of a staff doctor. Locum tenens contracts can last anywhere from a few days up to a year or more. Most agencies handle nationwide placements so it is a great way to go if you want to check out different locations before settling down. It is also a good way to gain additional experience – at a high rate of pay.

Join professional associations, such as the American Society of Anesthesiologists (ASA). On their website, you will find a virtual anesthesiology career center where members can browse exclusive job postings and meet with doctors and hospitals looking to hire anesthesiologists. Check back frequently as new jobs are posted every day.

Professional organizations are also very good for forming professional networking connections that could lead to career opportunities. They typically provide a calendar of events that may include workshops, conferences, seminars, and other activities where members gather. Networking is important in this career. Even small meetings provide a special opportunity to interact with established professionals. Remember, opportunities are often filled from the inside, without ever being advertised or listed on a job board. The only way to learn about them is to talk to people who may be in a position to know about them.

You can apply directly to hospitals, healthcare centers, and other potential employers in your area. You can send your résumé and cover letter whether or not there is an opening at the moment. However, your efforts will be more fruitful if you get some leads. Talk to other healthcare professionals and let them know what you are looking for. You may find that colleagues and acquaintances can refer you to a hospital that is in need of an anesthesiologist, as well as put in a recommendation on your behalf.

ASSOCIATIONS

■ **American Medical Group Association (AMGA)**
www.amga.org

■ **American Society of Anesthesiologists (ASA)**
https://www.asahq.org

■ **United States Medical Licensing Examination (USMLE)** http://www.usmle.org

■ **Association of American Medical Colleges (AAMC)**
https://www.aamc.org

■ **American Board of Anesthesiology (ABA)**
www.theaba.org

■ **American Board of Physician Specialties (ABPS)**
https://www.abpsus.org

■ **American Association of Nurse Anesthetists (AANA)**
https://www.aana.com

PERIODICALS

■ **Journal of Clinical Anesthesia**
https://www.jcafulltextonline.com

■ **Anesthesiology News**
www.anesthesiologynews.com

WEBSITE

GasWork
https://www.gaswork.com/search/Anesthesiologist/Job

Copyright 2019
Institute For Career Research
CAREERS INTERNET DATABASE

www.careers-internet.org

www.ingramcontent.com/pod-product-compliance
Lightning Source LLC
Chambersburg PA
CBHW071200220526
45468CB00003B/1099